The Complete Clean Eating Guide

Lose Weight Quickly, Achieve Optimal Health and Feel Energized with Clean Eating for Busy Families and Clean Eating Recipes

Emma Rose

Table of Contents

Introduction

I want to thank you and congratulate you for purchasing the book, *"**Clean Eating Guide**: Lose Weight Quickly, Achieve Optimal Health and Feel Energized with Clean Eating For Busy Families and Clean Eating Recipes"*.

This book contains proven steps and strategies on how to lose weight, have more energy, and stay healthy using the principles of clean eating.

There are so many different kinds of diet programs and products available in the market today and all you need to do is choose the one that you think will work best for you. If you do not want to try new products that helps you lose weight and boosts your energy, you should stick to something more basic and natural such as clean eating.

In this book, you will learn everything you need to know about clean eating. It is important to find out everything you can about this type of diet before you incorporate it in your lifestyle. You will learn about the benefits and principles of clean eating and some useful tips that can help you along the way. This book also includes some easy recipes that promote clean eating.

Thanks again for purchasing this book, I hope you enjoy it! Please take some time to stop by and LIKE our Facebook page:

https://www.facebook.com/joypublishing

With gratitude,

Emma Rose

Chapter 1

What Is Clean Eating?

You have probably come across the term 'clean eating' but you are still not familiar about its exact meaning. This is being used by people who work in the health and fitness industry such as personal trainers ad dietitians. People who are health conscious and workout fanatic also often use this word. Does it have something to do with cleaning the food before eating or cooking? Or maybe it has something to do with the kind of food that you eat.

The loose definition of clean eating is eating food in its most natural state. These days, people are starting to pay more attention to the kinds of food that they eat and how these foods are made. They take note of the food's ingredients and make sure that the food product only contains all natural ingredients.

The term clean eating first came out in the 1990s. Today, it is still being used by health conscious individuals from different backgrounds and culture to refer to the kind of all natural diet that they have. The definition of clean eating can vary from person to person. Some define clean eating as eating mostly fruits and vegetables while others define it as not eating anything artificial. You will find out more about these things as you read this book.

What Clean Eating is not?

If you think clean eating is another diet program, like the South Beach diet or Paleo diet, you are wrong because clean eating is a way of life. It also does not follow any strict rules about what food group to eat and not to eat, how many calories you should consume in a meal, and so on. This is the most basic way of healthy eating that promotes weight loss and boost energy.

Everybody can do this, even those who are not trying to lose weight.

Clean eating will not make you feel deprived or frustrated because it is so easy to follow. You do not even need to have a really strong determination because it is all a matter of choosing natural over artificial.

Is there such a thing as 'dirty' eating?

You are probably wondering if there is such a thing as 'dirty' eating or the opposite of clean eating. Clean eating does not literally mean eating foods that have less dirt. It means that you are choosing the best and healthiest food choices from different food groups in their most natural state. 'Dirty' eating is not the opposite of clean eating because there is no such thing as eating dirty. The opposite of clean eating is choosing the wrong food to eat and eating junk foods and processed foods that leave toxins in your body.

Clean eating also looks at the source of food. It should not come from large commercial manufacturers that use machines to process food. The foods that clean eaters usually use come from small farms that do not use chemicals and undergo processes. This is why clean eating is often associated with organic eating.

Chapter 2

Principles of Clean Eating

In every new diet program or plan, there are underlying principles that make up its foundation. These principles are the bases of the whole program or plan. Clean eating is not really a diet program but it also follows certain principles. Here are some of the basic principles of eating clean.

Eat Whole Foods

Whole foods are foods that are in their most natural state. This means that they have not been processed or tampered with in a factory or a laboratory. For example, the most natural state of an apple fruit is after you pick it directly from the tree. It becomes processed or tampered with when they extract juice from the fruit and add sweeteners and flavorings to produce ready-to-drink apple juice. On the other hand, homemade apple pies, apple marmalades, and apple cider are still good for clean eating because they are not processed in a factory and chemicals and artificial ingredients are not added. Whole foods come straight from the farm. Some examples include whole grains, fresh fruits and vegetables, unsalted nuts and seeds, and so on.

Avoid Processed Foods

Obviously, you should also avoid processed foods if clean eating involves eating only all-natural or whole foods. Processed foods have labels. You can see at the back of the food product that it has additional ingredients, preservatives, and other artificial substances to make the food last long and also to ensure that it tastes just like all the others. There are some foods that are processed in factories such as natural cheeses and whole grain pasta but these are not necessarily bad because they usually do not have artificial ingredients. The trick is to not buy any food item that has more than five ingredients or if the names of the ingredients are difficult to pronounce.

Do Not Use Refined Sugar

That fine white sugar may look cleaner than brown sugar but you should avoid this type of sugar because this has already been refined in the factory. Refined sugar has that sweet artificial taste which is so much different from the natural sweet taste of brown sugar. You should eliminate this from your diet because it only gives nothing but calories. To sweeten your food and drinks, you can use brown sugar or honey instead.

Combine Proteins, Carbs, and Good Fats

Some people who go on a diet make the mistake of removing one food group from their diet plan, such as carbohydrates, protein, or fat. This is not healthy because your body needs these nutrients. What you can do is to eat a balanced meal that has contains the right amount of protein, carbohydrate, and fats that your body needs. Combining these nutrients also make you feel more satisfied and full, which keeps you from snacking on junk food or eating more than what is necessary. This combination also gives enough fuel for your body to get you through the whole day.

Prepare your Own Meals

Instead of eating out, you should consider preparing your own meals at home. You should also consider packing your own lunch when you go to work. This is the best thing to do if you are planning to try clean eating because you know that the ingredients that you used to prepare the meal are natural and unprocessed. You should also avoid buying those ready-to-cook or instant meals in a box because these foods usually contain artificial ingredients. You can try some of the recipes that are included in this book.

Eat Smaller Meals

Instead of eating two or three large meals in a day, you should consider eating five to six smaller meals throughout the day to improve your metabolism and also to maintain that feeling of being full that will keep you from snacking on any food that you can find in the fridge or binge eating.

Avoid High Calorie Drinks

You should avoid high calorie drinks such as coffee or soft drinks because they add around 400 to 500 calories in a day, which is difficult to burn. Clean eating does not really require you to count your calories but it also does not mean that you can consume high calorie foods and drinks anytime you like. If you are thirst, you can drink water, unsweetened tea, or freshly squeezed fruit juice.

Chapter 3

Benefits of Clean Eating

Clean eating has a lot of benefits to your health. This is the reason why a lot of people want to try this way of eating. It is one of the key components of having a healthy lifestyle. Here are some of the more specific benefits of clean eating.

Improve Health and Wellbeing

Eating clean helps improve your health because you are eating all-natural food that does not have any artificial or chemical ingredients that are harmful to your health. Toxins from processed food cause diseases such as cancer, heart problems, and diabetes, to name a few. Clean eating also promotes a balanced diet because it encourages you to eat the right amount of nutrients. And if your body is getting all the nutrients that it needs, it will have a stronger immune system which protects your body against diseases. Your body will also feel lighter because you consume less meat plus you choose meat that has the best quality. Some people even completely forgo eating meat and get their protein requirements from other sources although this decision is all up to you. And because you are not eating meat, diseases that are caused by eating too much meat can also be prevented such as high blood pressure and stroke.

Aside from improving your physical health, eating clean also helps improve your mental health. This is because you are getting nutrients that your body needs which greatly improves your mood and feelings. It also helps prevent feelings of depression and anxiety.

Lose Weight

Clean eating also helps you lose weight because you are eating the right amount of food and the kinds of food that keep you feeling full. This is especially true if you are not eating a lot of meat because meat can contribute to weight gain. You do not need to try those expensive diet fads that become popular each year. You do not even need to make a lot of effort if you try clean eating. People who are not trying to lose weight shed extra fats and achieve their optimum weight without even trying after following the principles of clean eating. Clean eating also encourages you to eat five to six smaller meals in a day instead of three large meals. This method keeps you feeling full and satisfied throughout the day, which in turn keeps you away from snacks and sweets to satisfy your cravings and hunger pangs.

Boost Energy

People these days become exhausted easily because of their sedentary lifestyle. You often feel the slump after eating lunch. This can also be attributed to your unhealthy diet. If your diet consists mostly of refined sugar, you will have these dramatic energy spikes that tend to slow down in the afternoon making you feel lazy after lunch. If you change your diet and start eating clean, you will become more energized which in turn will make you more productive. And if you feel energetic, you will also be more inclined to exercise, which will further help you boost your energy, lose weight, and achieve good health.

Chapter 4

Tips for Getting Started

If this is your first time to try clean eating, you should learn some useful tips that will help you get started. These tips will make the transition from your old diet and eating habits to clean eating much smoother.

Define What Is Clean Eating For You

It has been mentioned in the previous chapters that the definition of clean eating varies from person to person. You need to have your own definition which will serve as your guide when buying food and preparing meals. The principles of clean eating are your basic guide but you can tweak them a little bit to better suit your personal needs and preferences. For example, one of the basic principles of clean eating is eating lots and lots of fruits and vegetables. If you like to add meat, you can do so because clean eating does not necessarily forbid you to eat meat. Just make sure that you are eating high quality lean meat.

Stock your Pantry with 'Clean' Foods

Now that you are starting this new way of eating, you should also do something about your pantry and your fridge which are most likely filled with processed food with artificial ingredients. Clean out your pantry and fridge by getting rid of food items that have artificial ingredients and that are obviously processed in factories. You can check the label and ingredients for this.

Once you are done cleaning out your pantry and fridge, you should now do your grocery shopping. Some may have a hard time coming up with a clean eating grocery list but it is actually simple. Just include lots of fresh fruits and vegetables and buy those products that have the word 'whole' in them such as whole wheat bread, whole wheat crackers, or whole pasta. Another keyword to look for is 'unsweetened' such as unsweetened almond milk, coconut milk, soy milk, and so on.

For food items that are difficult to find, such as a clean ketchup, you should consider making homemade ketchup using fresh tomatoes and other clean ingredients. It is important to prepare for the shopping trip especially if this is your first time by making a grocery list and doing a little research on food items that you can prepare yourself.

Give Yourself Time to Adjust

Transitioning from a lifestyle wherein you eat anything you like to a more disciplined eating habit like clean eating may be difficult for some, especially when they realize the amount of work involved in choosing the right kinds of food and preparing your own meals all the time. But once you get used to it and you started to reap the benefits of clean eating, everything will be so much easier. Just give yourself plenty of time to adjust. For example, you do not really have to give up all your favorite processed foods overnight such as pizza, cake, or doughnuts. You can still eat them while you are I the process of transitioning to clean eating. As you become accustomed to your new eating lifestyle, you can get rid of these processed foods one by one. You can find clean recipes of your favorite foods so that you can make them at home using clean ingredients.

These are the things that you need to know if you are planning to start a clean eating lifestyle. The next chapter includes some easy-to-make recipes that you can prepare for your whole family even when you are on the go.

Chapter 5

Simple and Easy Clean Eating Recipes

You will need some easy and simple recipes that you can whip up in just a few minutes if you are going to transition to a clean eating lifestyle. One great tip is to prepare your meals in big batches when you have free time and freeze small portions. This way, you and your family can just reheat the food whenever they need to eat. This will prevent you from eating out or eating just whatever is available. You might also want to invest in a cooler which you can pack with ice and take with you at the office or anywhere you go so that you can eat clean anytime, anywhere. You should also invest in a slow cooker where you can just leave the food that you are cooking while doing other things.

Here are some simple and quick clean eating recipes that are easy to prepare.

Cucumber and Tomato Salad

Ingredients:

- 2 medium-sized cucumbers, peeled and sliced thinly
- 2 cups cherry tomatoes, sliced in half
- ½ red onion, sliced thinly
- 1 tsp Dijon mustard
- 1 tbsp extra virgin olive oil
- 2 tbsp fresh dill
- 1 tsp honey (optional)
- Sea salt and pepper to taste

Procedure:

1. Combine cucumbers, tomatoes, and onion in one large salad bowl.

2. In a separate bowl, mix the remaining ingredients for the dressing using a whisk.

3. Pour the salad dressing into the vegetable mix. Toss to evenly coat the vegetables. Serve.

Roasted Salmon and Bok Choy

Ingredients:

- 2 8-oz salmon cut without skin
- 1 large bok choy, chopped
- ¼ cup white onion, chopped
- ¼ cup green peas
- ½ cup vegetable stock
- 4 tbsp butter
- 2 tbsp teriyaki sauce
- 2 tbsp olive oil
- ¼ tsp dried thyme
- 1 tsp sweet paprika
- Salt and pepper

Procedure:

1. Preheat oven to 375 degrees Fahrenheit.

2. Using a small brush, coat the salmon cuts with olive oil. Turn on the stove to medium heat and place a saucepan over the burner. Place the salmon on the saucepan, with the skin side facing down.

3. While one side of the salmon is cooking, use the same brush to apply teriyaki sauce on the top side of the salmon. Sprinkle a bit of salt, pepper, and paprika to season.

4. Put the salmon in the oven while it is still in the skillet and bake until the salmon is well cooked, which is around 15 minutes.

5. While waiting for the salmon to cook, steam the bok choy for about 10 mnuts or until they are properly cooked. You can also boil them, whichever you prefer.

6. Put a frying on the stove over medium heat and melt the butter. Add onion and cook for about five minutes or until translucent.

7. When the onion is cooked, add the veggie stock and the bok choy. Bring to a simmer.

8. Add the remaining ingredients which include the thyme and green peas. Sprinkle with salt and pepper to taste. Continue cooking until the liquid has evaporated, which is around 10 minutes.

9. Take out the salmon from the oven. Using aluminum foil, cover the skillet completely to allow the juices to evenly coat the salmon. Set this aside for about five minutes.

10. Put the bok choy on two separate plates and place the salmon on top. Serve while still hot.

Energy Booster Smoothie

Ingredients:

- 1 banana
- 1 cup raw oats
- 1 cup almonds
- 1 cup blue berries
- 1 tbsp chia seeds
- 1 tbsp ground flax
- 1 tbsp cocoa powder
- ½ cup plain greek yogurt
- 1 tbsp coconut oil
- A large drizzle of honey (the amount depends on how sweet you want it to be)
- A spoonful of homemade peanut butter
- Ice cubes

Procedure:

1. Put everything in a blender and blend until the mixture becomes thick and smooth, like a smoothie. Put in a pitcher and serve immediately.

2. This recipe includes a little bit of everything. The ingredients are quite flexible. You can substitute other clean ingredients if you do not have one or two of the ingredients above.

Blueberry Scones with Orange Zest

Ingredients:

- ½ cup frozen blueberries
- Zest of 1 orange
- 1 cup cashew flour
- 1 cup almond flour
- 1 cup coconut flour
- 1 tbsp hard coconut oil
- 1 ½ cups almond milk
- ¼ cup coconut sugar
- 2 tbsp baking powder
- a pinch of salt

Procedure:

1. Preheat oven to 400 degrees Fahrenheit. Get a baking sheet and line it with parchment paper.

2. In a large mixing bowl, combine the different kinds of flours, the baking powder, and salt and mix together using a spatula.

3. Cut the hardened coconut oil into small chunks using a fork and add this in your flour mixture. Mix together until the texture becomes crumbly. Add the orange zest and sugar and mix together using a fork.

4. Add the milk into the mixture and mix using a spatula.

5. Fold the blueberries into the mixture until they are evenly distributed throughout the dough.

6. Put the dough in your baking sheet lined with parchment paper and form a circle using your hands. The dough should be about 12 inches wide and an inch thick.

7. Once you are done shaping the dough, sprinkle the top with sugar.

8. You can use a knife to slice through the dough to make 8 scones. Do this as if you are slicing a pizza.

9. Bake the scones until the edges are brown and crisp, which is about 20 minutes, give or take a couple of minutes.

10. Once baked, take the scones out from the oven and set aside to cool.

11. You can separate the scones apart using a spatula or a knife before serving.

Slow Cooked Savory Soup

Ingredients:

- 1 large sweet potato, cubed
- 2 cups carrots, sliced
- 1 cup green beans
- 1 small onion, diced
- 1 clove garlic, minced
- ½ cup fresh cilantro, chopped
- 15 oz (2 cans) black beans in can, drained and rinsed
- 2 cups vegetable juice
- 2 cups vegetable broth
- ½ tsp black pepper
- ½ tsp red pepper flakes, crushed
- 1 tsp cumin
- 1 tsp chili powder
- Sea salt to taste

Procedure:

1. Put all the ingredients in a slow cooker. Cover the cooker with the lid and cook on low setting until the veggies are tender, which takes about 6 to 8 hours.

2. You can add about a teaspoon of cheese if you like.

3. You can also sauté the onion and garlic in olive oil before adding to slow cooker together with the other ingredients for a more subtle flavor.

4. You can also add about 2 cups of kale, coarsely chopped, at the last five minutes of cooking. Kale is also considered a superfood because of the amount of nutrients that it provides.

Turkey with White Bean Chili

Ingredients:

- 1 lb ground lean turkey
- 19 oz (1 can) white kidney beans, drained and rinsed
- 4 tsps chili powder
- 1 medium-sized onion, chopped
- 28 oz (1 can) whole tomatoes with juice, chopped
- 1 tbsp ground cumin
- ½ cup plain yogurt
- ½ cup water

Procedure:

1. Turn on the stove to medium heat and put a 12-inch skillet. Put the turkey on the skillet, adding salt for seasoning, and cook until the turkey is slightly browned, which is around 6 to 8 minutes. Continuously stir the turkey using a spoon to break it up into smaller pieces. Cook the onion in the same skillet for 4 minutes, and add cumin and chili powder. Cook some more for about a minute.

2. Add the beans, tomatoes with the juice, and water. Cook until the mixture is boiling. Reduce the heat to low and let it simmer without the cover for about 10 minutes. Serve the chili in bowls and top it with a spoonful of yogurt.

Quinoa Salad with Orange, Dates, and Asparagus

Ingredients:

For the salad:
- 1 cup raw quinoa
- ½ cup white onion, chopped
- I cup fresh orange sections
- 5 dates, pitted and chopped
- ½ lb asparagus slices, steamed and chilled
- ½ cup jalapeno pepper, diced
- ¼ cup pecans, chopped and toasted
- 2 tbsp red onion, minced
- 2 cups water
- 1 tsp olive oil
- ½ tsp sea salt

For the dressing:
- 2 tbsp lemon juice, freshly squeezed
- 1 garlic clove, minced
- 2 tbsps fresh mint, chopped
- 1 tbsp extra virgin olive oil
- ¼ tsp black pepper, freshly ground
- ¼ tsp sea salt
- Mint sprigs (optional)

Procedure:

1. For the salad: In a large non-stick skillet, heat the olive oil over medium heat. Sauté white onion for two minutes. Add quinoa and sauté for another 5 minutes. Add water and salt and bring the mixture to a boil. Once boiling, lower the heat and cover the skillet and let is simmer for 15 minutes. Turn off the heat and remove from the stove. Set aside for about 15 minutes to let the quinoa absorb the water. Put

the quinoa mixture in a large bowl and add the orange sections and the remaining ingredients. Mix gently.

2. For the dressing: Mix together all the ingredients, except the mint and mint sprigs, in a small bowl. Pour the dressing into the salad and gently toss until the dressing evenly coats the salad. Add the fresh mint and garnish with mint sprigs. Serve.

Black Bean Casserole

Ingredients:

- 15 oz (2 cans) black beans, drained and rinsed
- ½ cup vegetable broth
- 4 whole-wheat, low-sodium tortillas
- 1 cup shredded cheese
- 2 garlic cloves, minced
- 2 tbsp cilantro, chopped
- 12 oz unsweetened salsa
- ¼ tsp black pepper
- 1 tsp cumin
- 2 tbsp extra virgin olive oil
- Salt to taste

Procedure:

1. Preheat oven to 375 degrees Fahrenheit. Put skillet over medium heat and add olive oil. Saute garlic on the skillet before adding black beans and vegetable broth. Cook for three minutes. Add the spices such as cilantro, cumin, black pepper, and salt. Stir to evenly distribute the flavors.

2. Get an 8x8-inch casserole and spray with cooking spray. Put one tortilla on the dish, a quarter portion of the black bean mixture, a quarter portion of the salsa, and a quarter of cheese. Do the same steps until you have used up all the ingredients.

3. Once you are done layering the tortilla, black beans, salsa, and cheese, you should now cover the dish with aluminum foil. Put it in the oven and bake for about 20 minutes. You will know when it is cooked when the cheese becomes bubbly. Remove foil and put it back in the oven for another

8 to 10 minutes. Remove from the oven for the last time. You can add sour cream or Greek yogurt if you like.

Strawberry Cream Pie Parfaits

Ingredients:

- 1 ¼ lb fresh strawberries, sliced
- 1 cup whole-wheat flour
- 1 ½ cup ricotta cheese
- ¼ cup almond meal
- 3 tbsp raw honey, divided
- 2 tbsp safflower oil
- ¼ tsp sea salt
- 2 tbsp cold water

Procedure:

1. Preheat oven to 350 degrees F. spray an 8-inch square baking dish made of glass with cooking spray.

2. Combine almond meal, flour, and salt in a medium bowl using a whisk. Add safflower oil, honey, and cold water. Do not add these ingredients all at the same time. Be sure to stir the mixture until the ingredient is incorporated into the mixture before adding the next ingredient. The mixture will have a sandy texture, which is a little uneven.

3. Transfer the mixture into your baking dish and gently press with your fingers to ensure that the layer is even. Bake for about 21 to 24 minutes. Once the edges and bottom part are golden brown in color, take it out from the oven and let it cool.

4. Mix together honey and cheese in a bowl. You can use an electric mixer on high speed setting. Remove the crust from the baking sheet once it is cooled and place on a cutting board or any clean flat surface. Break the crust into bite-size pieces.

5. To assemble the parfait, you will need 6 parfait glasses. Divide the crust, strawberries, and cheese into six parts. Add your crust, cheese, and strawberries into the glass. Do this for all the other parfait glasses.

Crab Salad-Stuffed Eggs

Ingredients:

- 1 cup lump crabmeat
- 2 cups radishes, sliced thinly
- 8 large eggs
- 24 butter lettuce leaves
- 2 tbsp extra virgin olive oil
- 1 tbsp freshly squeezed lemon juice, divided
- 1 tsp dry mustard
- ¼ cup celery, finely chopped
- ¼ tsp ground black pepper
- 3 tbsps Greek yogurt
- ½ tsp salt, divided

Procedure:

1. In a large bowl, mix radishes, 1 tsp lemon juice, and salt. Cover with lid or plastic wrap and put it in the fridge for about 30 minutes.

2. Boil eggs in a medium saucepan. Be sure to cover the eggs with cold water. Once the eggs are boiling, reduce the heat and let it simmer for ten minutes. Turn off the stove and put the eggs in cold water to let them cool. Once the eggs are cool enough to hold, crack the egg shells and peel. If it is still a little too hot, you can peel the eggs under running water. After peeling the eggs, cut them in half vertically. Take out the egg yolks and put them in a sieve. You will need about 1 tbsp of yolks so set this aside.

3. In a medium bowl, combine the remaining lemon juice, ¼ teaspoon salt, pepper, and remaining egg yolks. Mix together using a whisk. Gradually add the oil while continuously stirring. Add the yogurt, crabmeat, mustard,

and celery. Gently stir until all the ingredients are well combined. Add salt and pepper to taste.

4. Create a fan using three lettuce leaves on each of the 8 plates. You should cut a very small part under the egg white to keep it steady. Add the crab filling into each egg white half. Each plate will have two egg whites. Add 1 tsp of egg yolk on top of the crap filling. Put the two egg white halves on one side of the plate and put sliced radish mixture on the other side. Do the same steps for all the remaining plates and ingredients.

Conclusion

Thank you again for purchasing this book!

I hope this book was able to help you to learn more about clean eating and how it can improve your health and well-being.

The next step is to start eating clean by following the guidelines that you have learned in this book. You should also try some of the quick and easy recipes included in the last chapter.

In addition, please remember to check out our Facebook page in order to find other resources and upcoming promotions:

https://www.facebook.com/joypublishing

With sincere thanks,

Emma Rose

Preview Of "Paleo Diet Guide for Beginners: Over 50 Paleo Diet Recipes for Fast Weight Loss and Optimal Health"

Introduction

I want to thank you and congratulate you for purchasing the book, *"Paleo Diet Guide for Beginners: Over 50 Paleo Diet Recipes for Optimal Health and Fast Weight Loss"*.

This book contains everything you might need to know when it comes to getting started with the Paleo diet. It is provided in an easily digestible format that allows you to better absorb the information. There are no complicated explanations about how it works! You'll be given what you need straight up so you won't have to waste time trying to understand exactly what the diet is. Whether it's for your overall good health or to lose a few pounds, Paleo can certainly help you with it. To help you get started, we'll do the same and start you off with 50 of the best Paleo recipes that you can slowly but surely shift your everyday menu to.

It's never easy changing a diet. I often fall into self pity when I can no longer have the foods I enjoy. Either I feel sorry for myself or I get rebellious and binge and anything and everything. I always knew the value of eating healthy. I could just never bring myself to do it. It wasn't until I had a miscarriage that I got serious about my health. I have made drastic changes that others just don't understand. But the pay off is the weight I've lost and the better health I'm experiencing.

My hope for you is not to be on another "diet." This isn't a restriction diet like Atkins. The goal is to have a lifestyle change. Lifestyle changes are more sustainable and maintain weight loss long term compared to restriction diets. The change is hard to start but worth it when you commit. The trick is to get the momentum to start.

Thanks again for purchasing this book. I hope you enjoy reading it and eating the recipes from it!

Chapter 1 – What Is the Paleo Diet?

The Paleo Diet is known by many names such as the cavemen diet, stone age diet and hunter-gatherer diet, to name a few. The concept behind this diet follows that of the Paleolithic era before the development of agriculture. Essentially, you consume the same foods that the cavemen used to eat. The focus is on eating food closest to its natural, unprocessed state. The cavemen would gather their food from any source available whether it was wild animals, berries, vegetables, or fruits. As a result, they were strong, fit, and healthy for thousand of years.

This type of diet is still very young, less than fifty years only, but more in depth researches and studies are being conducted to increase the information and knowledge on this diet. The results of previous studies conducted on the Paleo diet reveal the improvement of health to the people involved. This is attributed to the fact that no processed foods and additives are included. The Paleo Diet is a diet that works with our genetics – before machinery and processing got involved. Foods that were not available during the Paleolithic time such as dairy products, salt, sugar and grains are not included in the preparation of the Paleo diet.

The modern diet predominately consumed in the Western world is full of refined foods, trans fats, salt and sugar. These ingredients are known to indirectly cause diseases such as hypertension, diabetes, strokes, obesity and other heart problems. The list goes on even further with the increase diagnosis of cancer, Parkinson's, Alzheimer's, depression and infertility. "What an extraordinary achievement for a civilization: to have developed the one diet that reliably makes its people sick!" (Michael Pollen, Food Rules: An Eater's Manual, Penguin Books 2009).

Foods included in the Paleo Diet

- Fruit

- Vegetables

- Lean Meat

- Seafood

- Nuts/Seeds

- Healthy Fats (eg. coconut, avocado, nuts and seeds, olive oil, grass fed butter)

Foods NOT included in the Paleo Diet

- Dairy

- Grain

- Processed Food

Why not grain?

You may be surprised to see that grains are not included in the Paleo Diet. We are accustomed to grains being a part of a balanced diet. However, our bodies are not designed to deal with the nutritional components of grains such as gluten, lectin, and phytates.

Gluten is a protein substance found in wheat, barley and rye. Many people are discovering that their bodies are gluten sensitive and are eliminating gluten from their diet. The most extreme case of gluten sensitivity is Celiac Disease. Individuals with this disease can pick up the minutest trace of gluten and react immediately.

Lectin binds to insulin receptors and can also cause leptin resistance.

Phytates cause minerals to become unavailable during digestion.

Check out the rest of "Paleo Diet Guide for Beginners: Over 50 Paleo Diet Recipes for Fast Weight Loss and Optimal Health" on Amazon.

Or go to: http://amzn.to/1jIJUFX

Check Out My Other Books

Below you'll find some of my other books also available on Amazon and Kindle. Search for these titles on the Amazon website to find them.

Paleo Free Diet Guide for Beginners: Over 50 Paleo Free Recipes for Optimal Health & Fast Weight Loss

Paleo Desserts: Satisfy Your Sweet Tooth With Over 100 Quick & Easy Paleo Dessert Recipes & Paleo Baking Recipes

Raw Food Diet Guide: Lose Weight Quickly, Achieve Optimal Health & Feel Energized with the Raw Food Diet & Raw Food Recipes

Clean Eating Guide: Lose Weight Quickly, Achieve Optimal Health & Feel Energized with Clean Eating For Busy Families & Clean Eating Recipes

Alkaline Diet Guide: Lose Weight Quickly, Achieve Optimal Health & Feel Energized with the Alkaline Diet & Alkaline Recipes

Coconut Flour Recipes for Optimal Health & Quick Weight Loss: Gluten Free Recipes for Celiac Disease, Gluten Sensitivities & Paleo Free Diets

Almond Flour Recipes for Optimal Health & Quick Weight Loss: Gluten Free Recipes for Celiac Disease, Gluten Sensitivities & Paleo Free Diets

Wheat Free Diet for Beginners: Lose Weight Quickly, Achieve Optimal Health & Feel Energized with Gluten Free Recipes for Celiac Disease, Gluten Sensitivities & Paleo Free Diets

Detox Diet Guide: Lose Weight Quickly, Achieve Optimal Health & Feel Energized Through the 10 Day Detox

Sugar Detox Guide for Beginners: Lose Weight Quickly, Achieve Optimal Health, Feel Energized & Eliminate Sugar Cravings Naturally

Ketogenic Diet Guide for Beginners: How to Achieve Rapid Weight Loss, Optimal Health & Unstoppable Energy with Ketogenic Diet Recipes

Anti Inflammatory Diet for Beginners: Lose Weight Fast, Optimize Health, Slow Aging, Fight Inflammation, Conquer Pain & Increase Energy with the Anti Inflammation Diet Recipes

One Last Thing...

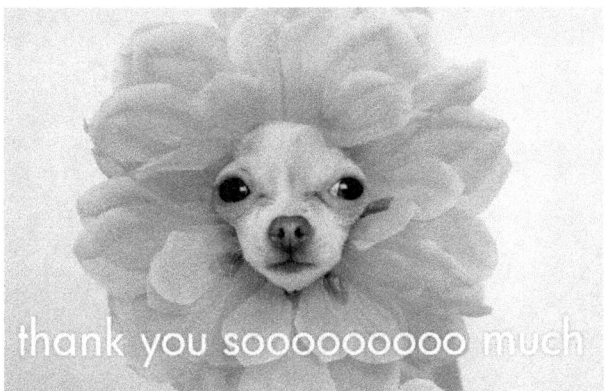

If you believe that this book is worth sharing, would you please take the time to let others know how it affected your life? If it turns out to make a difference in the lives of others, they will be forever grateful to you, as will I.

www.ingramcontent.com/pod-product-compliance
Lightning Source LLC
Chambersburg PA
CBHW070507290526
45790CB00003B/1136